About the authors

Jennifer Britt has been a journalist for the last ten years and is now the editor of *Natural Food Trader*. She has also contributed to *Here's Health* and *Alternative Medicine Today*.

Lesley Keen is a freelance journalist and PR consultant who specializes in health and alternative medicine. Trained as a journalist she has contributed to many newspapers and magazines such as *Here's Health*, *Alternative Medicine Today* and *Green Cuisine*.

Also published by Century

Aloe Vera by Frena Bloomfield
Jojoba and Yucca by Frena Bloomfield

FEVERFEW

Jennifer Britt and Lesley Keen

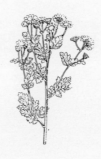

CENTURY

LONDON   MELBOURNE   AUCKLAND   JOHANNESBURG

First published in 1987
by Century Hutchinson Ltd, Brookmount House,
62–65 Chandos Place, Covent Garden, London WC2N 4NW

Century Hutchinson Australia Pty Ltd,
PO Box 496 16–22 Church Street Hawthorn
Victoria 3122 Australia

Century Hutchinson New Zealand Limited,
PO Box 40–086
Glenfield Auckland 10 New Zealand

Century Hutchinson South Africa (Pty) Ltd,
PO Box 337 Bergvlei 2012 South Africa

Photoset by Deltatype, Ellesmere Port
Printed in Great Britain by The Guernsey Press Co. Ltd,
Guernsey, Channel Islands

British Library Cataloguing in Publication Data

Britt, Jennifer
    Miracle plants: feverfew.
    1. Feverfew—Therapeutic use
    I. Title   II. Keen, Lesley
    615'.32355   RM666.F4/

ISBN 0 7126 1548 2

Contents

Acknowledgements

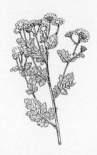

The authors would like to thank everyone who was so helpful in the research for this book and in particular:

Express Newspapers library staff
Dr Stan Heptinstall
Herbal Laboratories—John Grady, Sandra Crossley and Chris Thompson
Ann Jenkins
Stuart Lees
Jo Liddell of the British Migraine Association
Joan and Heather Linsley
Potters Herbal Supplies – David Hampson and Timothy Whittaker
Dr John Pugh
Dr Emlyn Roberts
Claire Swann
David Westcott

Introduction

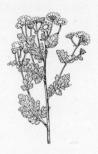

A young civil servant keeps it on her desk.

A bingo caller sings out its praises to seaside holidaymakers.

A Welsh doctor's wife and a Derby bus inspector have corresponded with people all over the world about it.

And thousands of people throughout Britain find a daily dose brings relief from the misery of arthritis, migraine and other ailments.

What is it?

It is feverfew – a herb which Plutarch wrote about many hundreds of years ago. It was popular during the Middle Ages, 16th and 17th-century herbalists gave much credence to its medicinal powers and it even earned itself the nickname 'the aspirin of the 18th century'. Now, after a period of neglect in which feverfew was regarded by most people as a weed which had a happy knack of invading their gardens, it is being hailed as an important modern medicine and scientists are busy finding out more about it.

In researching this book we have found that the Welsh have again and again played a significant part in bringing feverfew back into prominence. The publicity given to a Welsh doctor's wife who found relief from migraine and arthritis with daily feverfew sandwiches provoked huge public interest. One of the first feverfew capsules was made by a Welsh pharmacist from plants grown in his garden. A Welsh choirmaster in a village church told one of his choirboys about it – and that boy, Martyn Bailey, went on to become a scientist in the USA and he has carried out research on the herb.

More recently, a Welshman working in the Department of Medicine at University Hospital, Nottingham, took a plant into the laboratory and suggested that it should be studied as it was helping his uncle's arthritis. The researchers had heard about feverfew and its supposed biochemical actions and the work that they did on it was sufficiently important for the medical journal the *Lancet* to write a discussion piece about it. [1]

There are those who suggest that the taking of feverfew to treat migraine and arthritis simply has a placebo effect (the patient's faith in the herb fools the body into believing it is being helped) or that the taking of the herb coincides with the natural periods of remission which are a feature of both conditions. But we believe that the weight of evidence from people using feverfew, which is now backed by clinical and laboratory studies, shows that it really does work.

CHAPTER 1
Introducing Feverfew

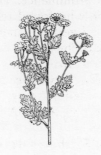

What is it?

Feverfew (*Tanacetum parthenium*) is a plant you have probably seen growing wild in your garden, in hedgerows or in areas of wasteland. It grows throughout most of Europe and has been introduced into the USA. A perennial plant with light green leaves which have a strong aroma, it grows to a height of around 2 ft and once established will seed itself each year. Flourishing particularly in a semi-shaded position in well-drained soil, it will, however, grow in virtually any conditions, producing white, daisy-like flowers from June to September.

Featherfew, featherfoil, flirtwort, midsummer daisy, nosebleed or bachelor's button: for an apparently unremarkable plant feverfew has a bewildering array of both popular and official names. The Welsh know it as wermod wen (white wormwood), referring to its bitter taste, and to the French it is *grande chamomille*. Over the years botanists have changed their minds when giving feverfew its official classification. Feverfew is part of the daisy or *Compositae* family, but it is the question of to which particular group or genus of the family it belongs which can prove confusing. You may see it referred to as *Pyrethrum parthenium*, *Leucanthemum parthenium* and *Chrysanthemum parthenium*. (The word *parthenium* refers to the species rather than the genus.)

The 17th-century English herbalist, astrologer and physician Nicholas Culpeper (1616 – 54) [2] described it as part of the *Matricaria* genus, but it has now been officially classified as one of the *Tanacetum* genus. Because the differences between each genus are small, it is easy to make a mistake and even nurserymen can be caught out. Sometimes some of the *Matricaria* family are sold as feverfew, including varieties named Snow Dwarf, Golden Ball and Tom Thumb. Their leaves may resemble those of *Tanacetum parthenium*, but their dome-centred flowers identify them.

There are different varieties of feverfew, including a double, ornamental one, but only one variety has been clinically tested. Dr Deborah Hylands, a research chemist in the Department of Pharmacy, Chelsea College, London, was one of the team which in 1985 published results of a clinical trial at the City of London Migraine Clinic using feverfew to treat migraine. [3] Writing in *Migraine Matters* in December 1984, she states that the wild *Tanacetum parthenium* is the only variety which scientists have subjected to chemical, clinical and pharmacological studies. [4] Dr Hylands describes how best to identify wild feverfew by examining the flower heads, which should have a flat, yellow centre, and by looking at the colour of the leaves. Leaf colour is important as there is a common variety, often called 'golden' feverfew, whose leaves are more yellow. She also points out that *Tanacetum parthenium* is said to be plastic, which means that its appearance may differ according to growing conditions. For example, leaves may sometimes be more or less serrated and the average size of the leaves may also vary.

Difficulties in identifying feverfew have even been a problem for manufacturers of today's feverfew remedies. Both German chamomile (*Matricaria recutita*) and tansy (*Tanacetum vulgare*) have been supplied to companies which have asked for feverfew. This emphasises the importance of laboratory testing of all supplies before the manufacturing process begins and the importance of obtaining the correct plant for anyone planning to eat the raw leaves.

Feverfew in history

References to the medicinal use of feverfew go back more than 1900 years to the first century AD when the Greek writer Plutarch offered a charming explanation of how the plant acquired the name *Parthenium*. He says it came about when a workman fell from the Parthenon in Athens during the construction of the temple and feverfew was used to save his life. The name feverfew is a corruption of the Latin *febris* meaning fever and *fugure* meaning to chase away, referring to the herb's use in treating fevers.

Throughout the centuries herbalists, who often mixed it with wine, honey or spices to help disguise the bitter taste, have had their favourite uses for feverfew. These fall into three basic categories: the treatment of fevers, headaches and migraine; women's problems such as regulation of menstruation, difficulties in labour and threatened miscarriage; and relief of toothache, stomach ache and insect bites and stings.

An anonymous herbalist, writing in 1525 in what became known as Bancke's Herball, [5] was an advocate of the 'toothache, stomach ache and stings' category. He called it

Federfoy and is quoted as using it for stomach troubles, cramp and also for insect bites and stings.

The English botanist and herbalist John Gerard (1545–1612) whose *Herball or General Historie of Plantes* was published in 1597, [6] recommends it for headaches and vertigo:

> Feverfew dried and made into pouder, and two drams of it taken with hony or sweet wine, purgeth by siege melancholy and flegme; wherefore it is very good for them that are giddie in the head, or which have the turning called Vertigo, that is, swimming and turning in the head. Also, it is good for such as be melancholike, sad, pensive, and without speech.

An astrologer as well as a herbalist, Nicholas Culpeper [2] saw a close link between herbs and the planets which he believed governed them—and naturally a herb governed by the planet Venus would be of special value to women. He says of feverfew:

> Venus governs this herb, and hath commended it to succour her sisters, women, and to be a general strengthener of their wombs, if the herb be boiled in white wine, and the decoction drunk; it cleanseth the womb, expels the after-birth, and doth the woman all the good she can desire of an herb . . . it is chiefly used for the diseases of the mother, whether it be the hardness or inflammations of the same, applied outwardly, or a decoction of the flowers in wine, with a little nutmeg or mace put therein, and drunk often in a day, is an approved remedy to bring down women's courses speedily.

He also recommends applying 'the boiled herb warm to the privy parts' or having the patient sit over the hot fumes of a decoction of the herb in wine or water. A decoction with sugar or honey could be used to cure chesty coughs and colds and was also recommended for cleansing the kidneys and bladder and getting rid of stones. He says:

> It is very effectual for all pains in the head coming of a cold cause, the herb being bruised and applied to the crown of the

head; as also for the vertigo. The decoction drunk warm, and the herb bruised with a few corns of bay-salt, and applied to the wrists before the coming on of ague fits, do take them away.

The distilled water taketh away freckles and other spots and deformities of the face. The herb bruised and heated on a tile, with some wine to moisten it, or fried with a little wine and oil, and applied warm outwardly to the places, removes wind and colic in the lower part of the belly. It is an especial remedy against opium taken too liberally.

In 1772 Sir John Hill MD [7], who wrote a family herbal, describes the use of feverfew like this: 'in the worst headaches this herb exceeds whatever else is known'.

Ancient herbal lore contained all kinds of rituals which must be observed when planting or gathering and these also applied to feverfew. The old sages said the name of the patient should be spoken out loud as the herbalist pulled the plant from the ground with his left hand and on no account should he look behind him while doing this.

CHAPTER 2
Re-emergence

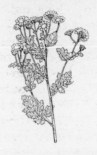

After being used for centuries to treat all kinds of conditions, feverfew fell into relative obscurity, together with many other traditional remedies, as the science of medicine advanced. Feverfew was still used by those familiar with traditional herbal remedies but it is only during the last decade that it has enjoyed a popular revival.

When the British Herbal Medicine Association was preparing the current edition of the *British Herbal Pharmacopoeia* feverfew did not even merit a mention as it was apparently not widely used by medical herbalists. When the book was published in its complete form in 1983 feverfew had already provoked sufficient national interest for the first commercial products to have come onto the market. Although it will almost certainly be included in the next issue it is still not a prominent herb in the medical herbalists' repertoire. Some herbalists are disinclined to use feverfew because they believe that it suppresses symptoms rather than attacking the root cause of the disease—the basis of their approach to healing.

However, many people continue to treat themselves with feverfew although manufacturers are unable to claim, on the pack or in literature, that feverfew products relieve migraine, arthritis or any other ailment. In order to make such claims, a manufacturer must obtain a Product Licence under the 1968 Medicines Act; new licences are not granted without evidence from long and costly clinical trials. Most herbal manufacturers are small concerns and say they are unable to afford research costing hundreds of thousands of pounds, which they could not recoup as a herb cannot be patented like a new drug product. So we can see that feverfew owes its return to popularity not to commercial 'hype,' but thanks to the many people who had heard about an ancient remedy and found it worked for them.

Migraine and arthritis sufferers who were already using feverfew long before the current publicity had perhaps initially experimented with it because of a friend's recommendation or because they had a recollection of granny keeping the plant at the bottom of the garden in case of headaches. Word of mouth and family tradition were the things which kept feverfew going. In 1978 a spate of publicity set it before an even wider audience. Ann Jenkins, a Welsh doctor's wife, had found relief both from migraine and arthritis through eating raw leaves and had been using it since 1974. Mrs Jenkins was featured on a Welsh television chat show and an article about her in *Prevention* magazine was followed up by the *Sunday Express* newspaper [8].

The *Express* article described how Mrs Jenkins used feverfew sandwiches to cure her migraine and how her friends and neighbours were astonished at the transformation in her health: 'Four years ago she looked so frail and ill that they wished there was something, anything they could do to help. But today Mrs Jenkins, an elegant woman in her late sixties, is full of health and energy and doing her best to help others.' The story attracted the attention of many people who were enduring migraine and arthritis and finding drugs ineffective or with unacceptable side effects. Soon after the publicity, Mrs Jenkins received the first of thousands of letters from people all over the world who wanted to learn more about feverfew. She has since done a great deal to promote the benefits of the herb by keeping up a massive correspondence and by writing about it—one of her articles about feverfew appeared in the *Welsh Medical Gazette*. This first major national publicity for feverfew has been followed by other occasional stories and articles in newspapers and magazines—often about people who had successfully used the herb or reporting on scientific investigations. Coverage has frequently amounted to little more than a few lines, but these passing references to the herb have served to introduce more and more people to it.

When the first article on Mrs Jenkins appeared in 1978, Derbyshire bus inspector, Ken Hancock, had already been studying feverfew for two years. He first came across it in a magazine article and friends had suggested that the herb might help to alleviate his wife's migraine. Mrs Hancock's migraines failed to respond to the herb but an unexpected side effect was relief of the mild osteoarthritis from which she was suffering. When she developed mouth ulcers, the most usual allergic reaction to the herb, she stopped taking it but her husband continued to grow feverfew and to supply local people. His involvement remained on this basis until 1984 when he wrote a letter to the *Daily Mail* about feverfew. He received 35,000 letters in a few weeks. Local papers followed up the story.

Mr Hancock estimates that he has corresponded with more than 50,000 people all over the world. An American manufacturer, Abco Laboratories, California, asked him to send them some germinated feverfew seeds. They have produced feverfew tablets using a freeze-drying technique and this new processing method means that feverfew seems to be taken without side effects. Mrs Hancock can now take feverfew to help her migraine and arthritis; from a situation where she suffered two migraines a week, she has suffered only one attack during her first seven weeks on feverfew. (The American product was not, at the time of writing, on sale in Britain.)

From the start Mr Hancock has been inundated with requests for information and for feverfew plants beyond the capacity of his own garden.

One of the alternatives he recommended were the feverfew capsules then being made by Dr and Mrs John Pugh of Cowbridge in Wales. Dr Pugh, a lecturer in pharmaceutical chemistry at the University of Wales Institute of Science and Technology, Cardiff, was running a part-time cottage industry growing feverfew and putting it into capsules. He is a pharmacist with a particular professional and personal interest in healing from plants. His introduction to the herb is an example of the way in which the word about feverfew was spreading. He first heard about it in North Wales where he discovered an old Welsh herbal which included a reference to wermod wen. He also heard the herb discussed by a Welsh language class which his wife was attending.

Using seeds from Mrs Jenkins' garden, Dr Pugh started to grow feverfew out of professional interest. He started to make capsules to help the migraine of a friend's son, but soon more and more people wanted his capsules, which he based on the 110–120 mg dose recommended by Mrs Jenkins. Although Dr Pugh is no longer producing capsules commercially, his professional interest continues through his university teaching job, where he has encouraged students to research the herb.

Modern folklore about the merits of feverfew drew it to the attention of other scientists, who examined the biochemistry of the plant. This led to larger-scale work to try to determine whether feverfew really is effective and, if so, how it works in the body. Scientists such as Dr Peter

Hylands of Chelsea College, together with research student Deborah Jessup, tried to find what was in feverfew which alleviated migraine. Research was building up evidence to show that there was a scientific basis for the claims made for feverfew. The City of London Migraine Clinic received an increasing number of inquiries about the herb and researchers came across so many patients who were treating themselves effectively with feverfew that they felt a closer examination of the herb was warranted, even if it was only to ensure that people were not doing themselves harm.

Medical journals had reported periodically on developments in feverfew research both at the City of London Migraine Clinic and elsewhere and the popular press had often picked up on these reports. But in 1985 two important studies were published—one by the City of London Migraine Clinic [3] and the other by a group in Nottingham. [9] The reports were published in the *Lancet* [9] and the *British Medical Journal* [3] and followed up in national and local newspapers and by BBC television on the *Tomorrow's World* science programme.

The first team to publish a report on feverfew was from Nottingham. Where scientists from the Department of Medicine at University Hospital and the Department of Haematology at City Hospital had found that in test tube experiments feverfew could be much more powerful in treating the symptoms of arthritis than the most potent drugs currently available. They called for more investigations into the herb to see if this success could be repeated in *in vivo* tests in patients. [9] This was followed by a report on a clinical trial at the City of London Migraine Clinic involving 17 patients over a period of several months in which their reactions to feverfew or to dummy capsules was recorded. [3] Again, it was discovered that feverfew appeared to have a soundly-based effect on migraine. The results of both these trials are examined in more detail later in this book.

Feverfew was now a sufficiently recognized treatment for migraine for the British Migraine Association to publish a leaflet telling members how to grow feverfew and how to dose themselves. Herbal manufacturers had also taken note of the popular and more technical references to feverfew and realized that there was a large potential market for commercially-produced preparations. Several companies started to investigate growing feverfew commercially to produce a supply of tablets or capsules. Potters Herbal Supplies in Lancashire had already examined feverfew in 1981, after a number of letters had appeared in the press praising its virtues as a remedy for migraine. Although feverfew had been neglected in herbal medicine, Potters were familiar with it and had used it in other products.

John Grady, the managing director of Herbal Laboratories, also based in Lancashire, read about the start of the City of London Migraine Clinic trials in the *Sunday Times* in 1983. He decided to launch a product using feverfew. Both Mr Grady and the directors of Potters were so convinced that feverfew would be an important and commercially successful medicine that they were prepared to overcome the major problem of supply difficulties. Herbal Laboratories had a product on the market in six months, and at about the same time another company, Weleda, came out with a homoeopathic feverfew. Potters followed with feverfew tablets in March 1984. There has since been a steady stream of new feverfew products in different strengths and forms—two being added to the list in the month that this book was finalized.

CHAPTER 3
Why Does It Work?

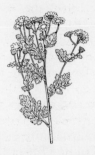

Feverfew is not a magic potion to be taken with the wave of a wand, a few medieval incantations and a generous helping of blind faith. For countless people over many centuries it has brought relief from pain and suffering and the scientists and doctors of today have found that it will work even in rigorously-controlled laboratory conditions. Considerable investigations have been carried out to find out exactly how and why feverfew works and a great deal of progress has been made, although there still seems to be a long way to go before the herb yields up all its secrets.

It is believed that the main active ingredient in feverfew is a group of chemicals called sesquiterpene lactones and these are the substances which have so far been the subject of the greatest amount of research. More than 500 of these chemicals have been identified in the plant kingdom, but they seem to be found chiefly in the *Compositae* (daisy) family to which feverfew belongs. Experts like Dr Stan Heptinstall, who led the Nottingham research team, believe that more work must be done to examine the sesquiterpene lactones in the herb and to look at other possible active ingredients.

Work on 'fingerprinting' chemical extracts of plants was carried out by a Polish group in 1978 [10] and they found that the sesquiterpene lactones were most abundant in tansy, balsamita and feverfew. Of the sesquiterpene lactones found in feverfew, a handful have been found to be pharmacologically active, the most significant of them being parthenolide. Parthenolide itself was first isolated from feverfew in the mid-1950s in Czechoslovakia.

A detailed study of the sesquiterpene lactones and other constituents in feverfew was reported in 1982 by Ferdinand Bohlmann and Christa Zdero of the Technical University of Berlin [11]. They found that feverfew contained a large variety of compounds, particularly in the stalk and leaves, the parts above the ground. Its elements included a very complex mixture of sesquiterpene lactones which were very difficult to break down into their individual components, especially as most were present in tiny quantities. They confirmed that parthenolide was the main constituent. However, scientists say there may be other substances whose degree of activity and efficacy will only be measured by further research.

One person who has taken an interest in feverfew is Dr Peter Hylands, lecturer in pharmacognosy at Chelsea College, London. Writing in Herbal Review in 1983, he described a study carried out at Chelsea College by Deborah Jessup (now Dr Deborah Hylands) as her PhD thesis. [12]

The study examined extracts of freeze-dried, powdered feverfew leaves for activity which could possibly play a role in migraine treatment. The lengthy process of dividing the substance into individual components eventually isolated some pure substances and, says Dr Hylands, these materials had 'intense biological activity and behaved in a way in the laboratory which led us to believe that they could be responsible for the efficacy of the plant. Some of the substances were new to science (they have never before been found in any plant)'.

So how do the active ingredients in feverfew work in the body? Feverfew works in a number of ways to achieve its effects. It has been described as the aspirin of the 18th century and it does seem to work in a similar way to aspirin by suppressing inflammation and affecting the size of blood vessels which cause pain in disorders such as arthritis and migraine. In a migraine attack experts believe that the blood vessels to the brain contract, reducing the blood supply, and then later they dilate producing the headache. At the earliest stage, before the pain begins, sufferers often complain of visual disturbances, difficulty with speech and even some tingling or loss of feeling.

The severe pain of migraine arrives with the production of substances called prostaglandins. These are among several substances produced to dilate the blood vessels and they are also concerned with prolonging and intensifying pain. These prostaglandins, together with other substances such as serotonin which influence dilation or constriction of the blood vessels, are formed when the platelets (tiny, disc-like bodies in the blood) aggregate, or clog together. This process releases serotonin from the platelets and also produces arachidonic acid, from which prostaglandins are formed. In further reading on migraine you may see serotonin referred to as 5HT (5-hydroxytryptamine). Serotonin can also be released during stressful situations.

Feverfew is understood to work at two stages during the chemical chain of events in a migraine attack, inhibiting platelet aggregation and the release of serotonin as well as the production of prostaglandins. Most drugs will only work at one of these stages. Reporting on feverfew trials at the City of London Migraine Clinic [3], Dr Hylands, Dr Stewart Johnson and their colleagues refer to the Chelsea College study, which found that as well as parthenolide the herb contains several new biologically active members of the sesquiterpene lactone group. Some of these, they say, make smooth muscle like blood vessels less responsive to substances including prostaglandins, serotonin and histamine which may cause the muscle to contract or dilate.

Migraine can be triggered by a number of factors. Tension and stress are the major causes, but dietary and environmental triggers are also common. Feverfew's effect on platelet aggregation is particularly interesting in the light of evidence to suggest that migraine is, in fact, a blood disorder, where the platelets show a greater tendency to clog together.

In October 1981 the *Lancet* published a report on a study by Edda Hanington and colleagues. [13] A total of 77 migraine patients and control subjects were studied and it was found that the platelets from the migraine sufferers showed a significantly higher tendency to aggregate during headache-free periods than those from control patients. The platelets from the migraine patients were markedly different in their behaviour and the researchers believed that this difference could explain the migraine attacks.

The scientists at Nottingham, reporting in 1985, [9] came up with some interesting results which threw new light on the possible use of feverfew in treating migraine, arthritis and psoriasis. They looked at the effect that feverfew has on the granule secretions of blood platelets—such as serotonin and the other substances implicated in migraine—and also the white blood cell secretions which are found in inflamed joints in rheumatoid arthritis. These white blood cell secretions, characteristic of arthritis, are produced by polymorphonuclear leucocytes which are granular white blood cells produced to gobble up bacteria, dispose of dead matter and release a potent bacteria-destroying enzyme. But these white blood cells can turn against the body itself and may be implicated in the tissue damage as in rheumatoid arthritis.

The Nottingham team concluded that feverfew was extremely effective in preventing the production of these secretions—more effective, in fact, than the type of drugs which are commonly prescribed to treat rheumatoid arthritis. These include aspirin and are known as non-steroidal anti-inflammatory drugs. In their report, the team said:

> It is clear that extracts of feverfew contain a material that is both water and lipid [fat] soluble that inhibits granule secretion. . . . The pattern of the effects of feverfew on platelet behaviour are, as far as we are aware, different from those that have been observed with more conventional inhibitors of platelet behaviour. . . . The extent of the inhibition of poly-morphonuclear leucocyte granule release by feverfew is much greater than has been achieved with high concentrations of non-steroidal anti-inflammatory agents.

But Dr Heptinstall stresses that it is important to remember that his team carried out experiments in test tubes and not in living patients. He says it is always possible that a substance which is seen to be effective in a laboratory experiment may not work in the body because it may never actually get into the blood stream if it is taken by mouth. However, results were sufficiently encouraging for him to set up three new clinical trials to test the effects of feverfew on patients suffering from migraine, arthritis and psoriasis. Although the initial research was able to suggest how feverfew may work in rheumatoid arthritis this may not be the same in osteoarthritis and the new tests will be examining both osteo and rheumatoid arthritis patients.

In a comment on the Nottingham study, the *Lancet* [1] says that feverfew's action in treatment of arthritis and psoriasis could be explained by its action in inhibiting the release of damaging materials from white cells in inflamed joints and skin. Its action on the release of serotonin by the blood platelets could account for its efficacy in migraine.

CHAPTER 4
Migraine

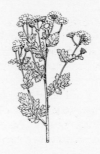

When you consider that the number of people in Britain suffering from migraine has been estimated at six million [14] it is not surprising that a natural substance which is able to help the majority of them should provoke such widespread interest. Doctors and scientists are also taking an interest in feverfew and those 'pioneers' who took their daily sandwich of raw leaves from the garden now find that their homespun remedy has a sound scientific basis.

The British Migraine Association, an organization founded and run by migraine sufferers which acts as a link between patients and the medical and research authorities, has taken a great interest in feverfew and supported research into the extent of its efficacy and safety. Although the Association does not actively promote feverfew—or indeed any other remedy—it does recommend it as a possible treatment for sufferers and one which for most people is without serious side effects. Since the Association was first alerted to the possible benefits of feverfew by Ann Jenkins in Wales, the herb has attracted a tremendous amount of publicity.

The Association's secretary, Mrs Jo Liddell, says that interest has been intensified as people become increasingly interested in alternative forms of medicine. All this has helped make feverfew fashionable, but, she says, feverfew has been proved to be genuinely beneficial and its popularity is not just a passing trend. Mrs Liddell sounds two notes of caution. First, feverfew will not help everyone and, indeed, in *The Dictionary of Modern Herbalism* [15], the president and director of research of the National Institute of Medical Herbalists, Simon Mills, says that it is the people who find their migraine is relieved through heat who usually find that feverfew will help them.

Results from the clinical trial carried out at the City of London Migraine Clinic [3] suggest that the herb may help 70 per cent of sufferers. Mrs Liddell, who is one of the 30 per cent for whom feverfew does not work, also points out that the herb can have side effects. When she tried it she found she was one of the people who suffered mouth ulcers, the most common adverse reaction. As secretary of the Association, Mrs Liddell is understandably cautious about recommending one particular remedy, especially as all the implications of its actions and ingredients have yet to be fully explored.

But a clear illustration of the interest in feverfew among migraine sufferers was shown by the number who responded to an appeal in the Association's monthly newsletter for volunteers to donate blood for use in further trials at the City of London Migraine Clinic. The relief that feverfew has brought to many migraine sufferers has been particularly welcome because so often they were the people for whom all other treatments had failed.

Evidence from trials

The British Migraine Association keeps in close touch with

the City of London Migraine Clinic and has helped to finance work there into the use of feverfew in treating migraine as well as other aspects of the problem. Writing in the Association's newsletter in 1983, Dr Stewart Johnson, former honorary research director at the clinic, said he first became involved with feverfew after seeing three patients who were taking it. The migraine charities were, he states, inundated with enquiries about feverfew and often these letters were passed on to him. However, he only became involved in clinical research after hearing from a doctor who was prescribing feverfew as a first course of action.

In an initial trial Dr Johnson surveyed 235 migraine sufferers who were taking feverfew regularly as a preventive measure. Seven out of ten of the patients, the vast majority of whom were taking feverfew in the form of fresh leaves, claimed that their migraine attacks were either less frequent, less painful or both as a result. The others found no relief. The success rate seemed almost unbelievable as orthodox treatments had not been very effective for these patients. But when he looked at the changes in the number of migraine attacks each month, the results were borne out. In fact one-third of the patients apparently had no further migraine attacks at all.

This work was followed by a double-blind placebo controlled trial in which the reactions of two groups were compared. This was carried out by Dr Johnson, with Drs Peter and Deborah Hylands and research assistant N. P. Kadam—with feverfew supplied by Chelsea Physic Garden. The results were published in the *British Medical Journal* in August 1985, [3] providing a dramatic boost for feverfew with evidence from clinical trials of its ability to bring relief to sufferers and it is interesting to look at this evidence in some detail.

Dr Johnson and his team invited 20 of the many migraine sufferers known to the City of London Migraine Clinic to be taking feverfew to participate in the trial. However, three of these patients were so worried that they might be placed in the placebo group that they did not take up the offer. The team wanted patients who had all suffered with migraine for at least two years with no more than eight attacks a month and who had been taking raw feverfew leaves each day for at least three months. They were anxious that the results obtained regarding feverfew should not be distorted because of drugs which the patients were taking at the same time. People taking drugs including tranquillizers, alpha blockers, beta blockers, antidepressants, non-steroidal anti-inflammatory agents of clonidine and pitzotifen were only allowed to take part if they had started to take the drugs before beginning self-medication with feverfew.

The trial took the form of a double blind, placebo controlled comparison between two groups of patients who had suffered from classical or common migraine for at least two years. These volunteers were chosen randomly to receive feverfew or identical placebo capsules. Patients were told to take two capsules every morning with food for six periods of four weeks and they were advised to treat attacks of migraine with soluble aspirin or their usual drug.

Patients kept diary cards on which they recorded the various symptoms such as visual disturbance, nausea, vomiting and headache. They recorded the times of onset and relief as well as details of any additional treatment and graded the severity of each symptom on a scale from one to three.

Nine patients were given placebo capsules and eight received capsules which appeared identical but which contained 25 mg of freeze-dried feverfew leaf. To ensure that patients were not aware of which group they were in, the placebo capsules were not only the same colour as the feverfew, but also smelt the same as the contents of each bottle was sprinkled with a small amount of feverfew powder.

Both the active and placebo groups had been taking about the same amount of feverfew each day before the start of the test. The active group had taken an average of 2.44 leaves per day and the placebo group slightly less with 2.33 leaves. On average the placebo group had been taking feverfew a little longer than the active group. For both groups feverfew had reduced significantly the frequency of migraine attacks, though the average for the active group before starting to take the leaves was much higher than that for the placebo group—7.44 attacks per month compared with 3.94. Once they had started to dose themselves with feverfew the active group found they had only 1.63 attacks each month and the placebo group 1.22, so at the start of the study the average frequency of attacks was similar for both groups.

Patients taking the dummy capsules reported more frequent headaches and other symptoms than those on the real thing and two of them found their migraines returned with such severity that they were forced to drop out of the trial and start taking feverfew again. The team reported that once back on feverfew their condition improved. One of the patients who dropped out also reported disturbed sleep and stiffness in joints in the mornings while taking part in the trials and was not prepared to tolerate these additional symptoms.

Results were compared after the first three months and over the whole of the six-month trial and these showed that while the feverfew group kept their level of migraine much the same as it was when they were on self-medication, the placebo group's records showed that they had regressed to the levels experienced before they began taking feverfew. Those on feverfew reported an average of 1.5 attacks a month during the last three months of the test and an average of 1.69 over the whole six months. Those in the placebo group suffered 3.43 attacks a month in the final three months and an average of 3.13 over the six months. Not surprisingly, most patients, when asked, were able to guess correctly each month which group they were in.

As well as reducing the frequency of migraine attacks, the feverfew also seemed to have a significant effect on the nausea and vomiting which often accompanies an attack. Those in the feverfew group found only 42 per cent of attacks were accompanied by these symptoms compared with 79 per cent in the placebo group.

Everyone in the placebo group reported at least one adverse event during the trial, but only four of the feverfew group reported them and two of these were said to be stiffness or pain in the joints which the patients had always had. The other adverse events reported were colicky abdominal pain, palpitations and slightly heavier periods. In the placebo group there were five reports of nervousness, jumpiness or tension, three of tension or non-migraine headaches, two of disturbed sleep, three of new pain or stiffness in joints, two of tiredness and one each of nausea, lighter or irregular periods and slightly heavier periods.

In discussion of the trial, the researchers said they believed these effects constituted a genuine post-feverfew syndrome when 164 users, who had ceased taking the herb had been asked to describe their symptoms, about one in ten complained of moderate to severe aches, pains and stiffness in joints and muscles as well as anxiety and poor sleep.

The team also said that the dried feverfew capsules did not appear to affect 'blood pressure, heart rate, body weight, or the results of haematological and biochemical tests'.

What the users say

Mrs Ann Jenkins, the Cardiff doctor's wife who has done so

much to introduce other people to the benefits of feverfew, first started taking it herself in 1974 when a friend suggested that she should try a plant which was growing in a relative's garden and which was supposed to be 'good for most things'. Mrs Jenkins did some research to establish just what this plant was and, having discovered it was feverfew, she decided to give it a try. She had suffered from migraine since adolesence and when she started taking feverfew she was suffering so badly that she was spending two days out of every eight or ten in bed. The pattern with her migraine was that after the first day of pain she felt very sick. She had taken all kinds of medication but experienced no lasting relief and some adverse side effects.

At that time there were no commercially available feverfew tablets, capsules or essences, certainly none of which Mrs Jenkins was aware, and she began to take raw feverfew leaves at the rate of three small leaves or one large leaf per day in a sandwich, sometimes with a little honey. 'It took six months for the sickness to stop and then another month and the migraines stopped altogether,' said Mrs Jenkins, who still finds that the fresh feverfew works best for her. She has not suffered a migraine in the last 13 years, but she says that she does sometimes experience an aura (the initial symptoms of a migraine before the pain begins) when fresh leaves are not available and she is taking the dried herb.

Mrs Jenkins had been receiving hospital treatment for osteoarthritis and in common with many other people taking feverfew, she found that it had beneficial side effects. 'Although originally I took feverfew for migraine, I realised afterwards that my arthritis was getting less and less,' she said. After about ten months on feverfew her arthritic symptoms disappeared. 'Really I have a new lease of life. Over the last ten years I have been doing work I could not possibly have done before,' she said. Mrs Jenkins estimates that she has been in correspondence with 2–3000 people throughout the UK and overseas concerning the benefits of feverfew and it seems that those who find relief by using the herb are keen to spread the word to help others.

Here are some of the experiences we came across in researching and compiling this book.

Two migraines a week were a way of life for a little boy called Bruce, who was diagnosed as having migraine when he was just six years old. Bruce, who is also hyperactive, was seen by specialists, but they could find no physical illness to explain his problems. Bruce's mother then became a vegetarian and she first heard about feverfew at the local health food shop. The first product she tried failed to give Bruce any relief from his migraine attacks, but a second attempt with a 125 mg tablet had an immediate effect. His attacks dropped from two per week to one a month. His father said the improvement 'obviously made Bruce much happier and because of this he had hardly any time off school. This wonderful herb has certainly helped him'. Now his father has passed on the message to countless holiday-makers from the stage of the seaside theatre where he is resident bingo caller.

Mr H., a 38-year-old communications manager, was diagnosed as suffering from migraine in 1981. He took various painkillers with no effect at all and at the time he started taking feverfew he was on six migraine-preventive tablets a day. He heard about feverfew through health and homoeopathic magazines and decided it was worth a try. He takes feverfew essence once a day as a preventive measure and says that if he feels a headache coming on a teaspoonful of feverfew essence placed under the tongue usually does the trick. 'It can be repeated every hour or so, but I advise you to wash it down with plenty of sweet tea—it tastes awful!' he says. Headaches that come on when he does not have any essence available are best dealt with by using tablets which are easier to carry around.

From suffering one migraine a week before taking

feverfew, Mr H. now reports only one every six months. He attributes this to feverfew, accompanied by a change in diet. He has cut out chocolate, cheese, yeast and beef extracts and all fatty dairy produce. His intake of preventive drugs is down to two tablets a day and he hopes to reduce this even further.

Mr K., a retired head teacher in his mid-50s had been taking a proprietary migraine relief capsule recommended by a pharmacist to ward off the infrequent attacks he had suffered for over 30 years. He found the capsules effective, curing the attack within 15–30 minutes if he was able to rest in a darkened room, but pressure of work had led to frequent migraines during 1985 and his neighbour, who had studied herbal remedies, suggested that feverfew may help. He started taking one small leaf whenever he felt an attack coming on. He says that relief was almost immediate, certainly within moments, with no side effects and he feels better more quickly with feverfew than with the capsules from the chemist.

Mr F. is a 32-year-old insurance agent, whose migraine attacks were diagnosed in 1973. He tried many different pharmaceutical drugs, some of which had no effect and others which worked for a short time until he appeared to become immune. A friend of his mother suggested feverfew and in May 1985 he started taking two small fresh leaves each morning. He says it seemed to reduce the attacks immediately without any side effects. He continues to take feverfew 'as regular as clockwork' and he now keeps potted feverfew plants indoors to minimize the risk of being without it during the winter.

Miss R., a 20-year-old civil servant, was diagnosed as suffering from migraine in June 1983 and started taking a proprietary migraine relief product and then a prophylactic from her doctor. The first had no effect and the second caused drowsiness and she said that although she did not always get a headache, she did experience particularly distressing 'aura' symptoms, including dizziness, visual disturbances, sickness, diarrhoea and limb cramps as well as some blackouts. Even if the headache did not then develop she was left exhausted for the rest of the day.

When she found that the tablets did not bring relief, she tried to amend her diet and finally her doctor told her nothing more could be done and she would have to put up with the distress. She learnt about feverfew after her mother heard a talk from a local woman who had studied herbal remedies and since starting to take one leaf every day she has had no migraine. She even keeps a feverfew plant on her office desk.

Mrs M. is a 79-year-old housewife who has been suffering migraine attacks over a long period. She says she found almost immediate relief when she started to take feverfew, which she had heard about from a friend. She started to take it when her daughter obtained a supply of tablets from a health food shop. She says that since she has been taking one tablet a day she has had only an occasional attack. 'I would recommend them without hesitation,' she said.

Mrs S., aged 54, had suffered from time to time with severe migraine and found that the attacks were gradually becoming more frequent so that she was waking with the symptoms nearly every Sunday and the pain was persisting all day. Doctors, medicine and injections had not helped. Feverfew was suggested as a possible course of treatment by a health food shop and Mrs S. started taking one tablet per day. In the first month she reported two 'mini-migraines' and in following months none at all. 'I have been completely free of migraine and life has taken on a new look,' she said.

Mrs L. had suffered from migraine for 20 years and said she had lost count of the many remedies she had tried. Within three months of starting to take feverfew capsules, she said she was able to eat cheese and chocolate again and had experienced no attacks at all. 'I used to have at least one migraine every two weeks, sometimes the attacks were more frequent but I really do believe that I am cured,' she said.

CHAPTER 5

Arthritis and Other Ailments

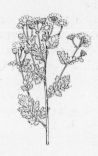

Arthritis

While the overwhelming concentration of interest in the media has focused on the benefits of feverfew in treating migraine, it is believed that even more people are taking it to obtain relief from arthritis. As we have already seen, some patients taking it for migraine have found that a welcome side effect has been relief from arthritic aches and pains. Feverfew has undergone trials to examine its efficacy in migraine but similar experiments in regard to arthritis were only at the planning stage at the time of writing this book.

Osteoarthritis and rheumatoid arthritis sufferers are among those who find feverfew beneficial and it is thought that the herb relieves inflammation. There is also evidence to suggest it may even help prevent the process which leads to the inflammation in the first place.

Commenting on the Nottingham trials, the *Lancet* said that when feverfew was mentioned in a daily newspaper 25,000 requests for further information were received.

'This suggests that if general practitioners, neurologists, rheumatologists and determatologists asked their patients about non-prescribed medication they would find that many of them were consuming feverfew.' [1] *The Lancet* went on to say that the scientists in Nottingham had discovered a new and powerful way in which feverfew was working and this could explain its success in treating arthritis and migraine.

It is clear that medical and scientific examination of feverfew and its efficacy in treating arthritis is still at a very early stage and much more work needs to be done. An estimated twenty million people experience some form of rheumatic pain every year, including eight million who seek medical advice [16] so there should be no shortage of patients willing to testify to the relief that they have experienced by taking the herb.

What the users say

Joan Linsley of County Durham was introduced to feverfew by her grandmother, who was a matron in a Victorian school. Joan gave little thought to the herb until 1974 when she found her mobility becoming increasingly restricted through osteoarthritis. Since then a small dose of feverfew has become part of the daily discipline which has given her a virtually pain-free life. She now grows feverfew both for herself and for other local people who have heard of its usefulness.

Joan recalls that in her Surrey childhood in the 1920s her grandmother kept feverfew in the garden and took it whenever she felt a headache coming on. 'She used to send me and my sister down to the end of the garden to pick some of the plant when she started to feel the pain,' she said. As well as being knowledgeable about many herbal first-aid remedies, her grandmother was a great believer in eating well to keep healthy and Joan admits that she had paid little attention to diet and was eating too much junk food. Her arthritis reached the stage where she sometimes had to be carried to and from the car and on occasions resorted to crawling upstairs.

For six years Joan had taken an anti-inflammatory drug which deadened the pain sufficiently for her to 'hobble about' but she was concerned about long-term effects and becoming dependent on the drug and decided to try an alternative approach. A diet in which red meat and sugar took a back seat and wholemeal foods, fresh fruit and vegetables were to the fore was one part of her recovery plan. A daily dose of a tiny leaf of feverfew—about the size of a large thumbnail—was another vital part of her intake. She also stresses that a positive attitude is important. She now finds it difficult to recall the terrible pain she used to suffer and has only the occasional twinge to remind her of her arthritis. The woman who once had to go upstairs on her hands and knees is now able to walk for miles and ride her bicycle.

Miss A., a 74-year-old retired teacher was diagnosed as having arthritis in her right hip in 1979–80. She took various drugs but said that side effects and lack of pain relief caused her to abandon them. She heard about feverfew in autumn 1985 from a friend who had a particular interest in herbs and gave her a health magazine to read. She started by taking feverfew essence and then moved on to the herb in tablet form. After about six weeks she experienced relief from pain. She is still taking feverfew tablets and has been able to reduce the dosage. 'I have experienced great relief from feverfew. I was almost on my knees but can walk fairly well now. I have recently had a flare up, but I think this was due to the cold weather and the fact that my heating packed up,' she said.

Mrs R. is a 66-year-old retired dancing teacher and writer who was diagnosed as having osteoarthritis. She took many conventional medications such as cod liver oil, aspirin and heat treatment with fair results but she found she experienced regressions. She decided to start taking feverfew when she read about it in a newspaper in 1983. She takes five drops of essence three times a day, with occasional 'rests' of two to three weeks. She says that within four days of starting to take feverfew she experienced some pain relief and was sure it was doing her good after two or three weeks and she says her doctor has been impressed by the pain relief she has gained.

Mr L., a 77-year-old retired man, has suffered from osteoarthritis since 1978, with an operation to remove a knee cap in 1980 and to replace a hip joint in 1984. He read about feverfew in the *Daily Mail*, which published a letter about it in 1983 and started to take capsules at the rate of one a day. The feverfew has brought him great relief from pain, with the first benefits felt within three days of starting treatment. Mr L. continues to take feverfew capsules during the winter, discontinuing them when supplies of fresh leaves are available from the plants he grows in his own garden. He either eats the leaves or drinks an infusion.

Mrs C., an 82-year-old housewife, began to suffer from pain in a hip joint early in 1985 and heard about feverfew from a friend. She started to take one tablet a day in April of that year and found relief after four weeks. She continues to take the tablets and says she has recommended it to a number of other people.

Mrs M., writing to one of the manufacturers, said: 'The heat has gone out of my knees and ankles, consequently I am sleeping well and feeling much better.'

Psoriasis and skin troubles

The team of scientists in Nottingham [9] suggest that the way that feverfew works in psoriasis is similar to its effect on rheumatoid arthritis. Its ability to inhibit the release of damaging materials from the white blood cells seems to apply to the inflamed skin of a psoriasis sufferer as it does to the joints of someone with arthritis.

Feverfew has also been used to good effect in treating eczema. Joan Linsley decided to try it on her daughter Heather, who had persistent eczema. Heather was 13 when she first started taking one small feverfew leaf daily in a sandwich. She found that the eczema, which was mainly on her hands, responded quickly to the herb. The condition flared up again when Heather started picking the feverfew out of the sandwiches because she did not like its bitter taste. Once she went back to the herb her eczema became manageable again and she still takes a small dose about three times a week.

Perhaps the time will come when feverfew ointment will be more widely available and external application will heighten the effect of the herb taken internally.

In an article in *Herbal Review* in 1980, Dr Elizabeth Woodward describes how a decoction of feverfew can be applied externally. [17] She finds it effective in helping to heal ulcers, wounds, conjunctivitis and scalp disorders. She also says that it is sometimes used to brighten fair hair. In Culpeper's day the distilled water of feverfew was also used cosmetically to get rid of freckles, spots and 'other deformities of the face'. [2]

Childbirth, menstruation and allied problems

Gynaecological problems were among the main uses to which Culpeper put feverfew. He advocated it in many different forms. To promote menstruation he used it applied outwardly or as a decoction of the flowers in wine with the bitterness disguised by nutmeg or mace. He used a decoction with water or wine when the patient would sit over the hot fumes 'and some cases to apply the boiled herb warm to the privy parts'. He prescribed it as a decoction boiled with white wine to cleanse the womb and expel the afterbirth.

Rather more up to date, in the *Dictionary of Modern Herbalism* [15] Simon Mills confirms feverfew as a uterine stimulant and says it can be used in cases of sluggish menstrual flow and congestive dysmenhorrhoea (period pains). There is evidence to show feverfew's ability to inhibit the production of certain prostaglandins. It is interesting to note that in cases of dysmenorrhoea it is the production of prostaglandins which causes the contractions which, if they are severe, cause pain. Other painful menstrual symptoms, like nausea, vomiting, diarrhoea and headache may be the result of prostaglandins causing contractions in the smooth muscle of the stomach, intestines and blood vessels in the brain.

Feverfew's use as a uterine stimulant also links it with a traditional use as an agent for inducing abortion. The flowers in particular have been used throughout Europe in folk remedies to induce abortion as well as promote menstruation.

In the 1985 study at the City of London Migraine Clinic, reported in the British Medical Journal, [3] one of the adverse effects noted by one of the feverfew group was slightly heavier periods. Among the placebo group there was one similar report and another which spoke of lighter or irregular periods, though this may be attributed to a post-feverfew syndrome or withdrawal symptoms.

Tension, nervousness and insomnia

Both Gerard [6] and Culpeper [2] advocated feverfew for depression. Gerard used it powdered and taken in honey or sweet wine and Culpeper used it with wine. This use of feverfew is confirmed by a man who came across it regularly in his Yorkshire childhood and who still takes it to treat migraine. He says: 'I can remember in my youth it was not uncommon to see people scouring hedgerows looking for various plants to use in medicines or cooking. My grand-mother was very interested in herbs and feverfew was one of the things she used to give to you if you were het up.' One unusual use to which she put the herb, which grew wild in the area, was as a salad ingredient.

Again, in the City of London Migraine Clinic trial, [3] the nine patients in the placebo group reported five instances of nervousness or tension, three of tension or other headaches and two of insomnia or disturbed sleep patterns. Dr Johnson and his colleagues say this is due to post-feverfew syndrome, but when in another study, 164 people who had stopped taking feverfew were asked to describe their symptoms only one-tenth of them complained of aches, pains and stiffness in joints together with central nervous system symptoms of anxiety and poor sleep.

Hay fever

Relief of this tiresome seasonal complaint is one of the side benefits which some people experience when taking fever-few for migraine or arthritis. Ann Jenkins says she knows of several people who have successfully taken the herb to ward off the sneezes, streaming eyes, headaches and general stuffiness which can make summer a misery. One person who tried the remedy on her recommendation was a 23-year-old student from Cardiff, Miss T., who had suffered from hay fever since the age of three. With her university final examinations due in summer 1985, her mother encouraged her to take a regular dose of feverfew over several months before the start of that year's pollen season. For the first summer in twenty years, she was not troubled by nasal swelling, catarrh, sneezing and headaches. She admits that it might have been coincidence that her symptoms disappeared the summer she tried feverfew but she continued to take doses of the herb in anticipation of another summer free of hay fever.

Vertigo

Culpeper [2] and Gerard [6] agree that feverfew is effective against vertigo. Gerard used powdered feverfew in honey or sweet wine and Culpeper says: 'It is very effectual for all pains in the head coming of a cold cause, the herb being bruised and applied to the crown of the head; as also for the vertigo.'

Simon Mills, writing more than three centuries later, speaks of its uses in treating conditions such as vertigo, tinnitus and other problems in the head where the patient can find relief through heat.

Insect bites

Bancke's Herball [5] talks of the use of feverfew to treat insect bites. In the article 'Feverfew Faces the Future', *The Pharmaceutical Journal*, May 1984, [18] Dr Mike Berry, senior lecturer in pharmacognosy at Liverpool Polytechnic poses the question of whether feverfew's anti-histamine properties [in inhibiting the release of histamine in the body] could be linked with its recorded uses for insect bites.

Feverfew was also used in the Mediterranean as a folk remedy to repel insects by scattering the dried flower heads on the floor. We came across a tale from a pharmacist and herbalist which suggests that there may be some sound basis for using it as an insect repellent. Marjorie Robinson is a member of the British Herbal Medicine Association's scientific committee and her husband is a former secretary of the Association. They were first alerted to the increasing current use of feverfew when a women's magazine wrote about the herb and included their address as a source of information. Although Mr and Mrs Robinson, who are both in their seventies, had no need of feverfew medicinally, they did try it out as an insect repellent. For two years they planted feverfew together with their broad bean seedlings in the vegetable garden and found that, unlike their neighbours, the beans were completely free from black fly one year and suffered hardly at all in the following year. 'If we get results like this again we will consider it really does work', said Mrs Robinson.

Many of the uses recorded for feverfew concern serious ailments and therefore anyone taking or considering beginning a course of feverfew should discuss it with their doctor, particularly if they are receiving any other medication.

CHAPTER 6
Dosage and Contra-indications

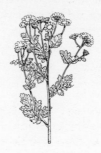

Who should not take feverfew?

Although feverfew has been in wide use for centuries it has not been subjected to the full battery of modern tests for toxicity and other effects. It is therefore sensible for some potential users to think carefully about taking it. It is important to remember that plants used in herbal medicine can be very powerful and as much care should be exercised in taking these natural remedies as a patient would use when taking pharmaceutical drugs.

Certainly, in view of its association with gynaecological treatment, including expulsion of the afterbirth, induce-ment of menstruation and its ancient use in provoking abortion in cattle, it is wise for pregnant women to avoid it. Feverfew should also not be given to babies, children or breast-feeding mothers.

Results of trials to test whether feverfew could cause mutation of cells or contribute in any way to causing cancer were not available at the time of writing and until evidence is available, cancer patients should treat the herb with caution.

People already taking drugs should consult their doctor before taking feverfew. It has been suggested that feverfew may lower high blood pressure so anyone taking drugs for this condition would have to be very careful.

The British Migraine Association has dealt with numerous inquiries about feverfew in recent years. The secretary, Jo Liddell, says that she has to stress repeatedly the power of feverfew, warning that the last thing people should do is to 'eat it like spinach'. She says 'I have had to write to so many people explaining that because it grows in your garden it does not mean it is not a drug. It is a drug and it is a very strong one'.

The leaf eaters

Feverfew preparations have only been available commercially fairly recently. There are still many people who use the traditional methods of eating fresh leaves from home-grown plants and preserving the herb for use when the fresh leaves are not available. This seasonal shortage was recognized by Culpeper, who advises 'If the herb cannot be got in winter; a syrup of it may be made in summer'. It was also used in its dried and powdered form by the old herbalists.

The taste of feverfew is very strong and bitter. Many people who find fresh leaves the most effective form make it more palatable by eating it in a sandwich with another strong-tasting substance such as honey, sugar or salad cream to disguise the bitterness. Honey can also be used to preserve the dried herb.

Leaves to be eaten raw should be freshly picked. It is suggested that when growing feverfew for home use, three plants should be maintained – two to set seeds for new supplies and one to crop daily. The plant being used medicinally should not be allowed to flower.

How much should you take?

There seem to be no firm rules for dosage of either raw leaves or commercial preparations. The leaflet issued by the British Migraine Association on feverfew and migraine advises 'one large or three smaller leaves' a day and says a small leaf is one measuring about 3 cm by 3 cm. Mrs Jenkins recommends one large leaf measuring 3½ in × 3 in or three smaller leaves (2 in × 1¾ in). She says this should be taken preferably between meals or at bedtime. This dosage works out at 127.5 mg of dried and powdered feverfew. However, some people find that they can control symptoms effectively with smaller doses; others require more.

Commercial preparations vary from homoeopathic preparations to 250 mg capsules and even among herbalists there is room for discussion on dosage. The City of London Migraine Clinic project [3] demonstrated how different people respond to different doses of feverfew, just as they do with conventional drugs. Patients taking part in the study were instructed to take two 25 mg capsules of feverfew daily. This dosage was arrived at after examining the amount of raw feverfew that those taking part had been consuming. The average worked out at about 60 mg and dosage was fixed at 50 mg a day.

One man taking feverfew capsules found that this dose did not seem to be enough. Although his headaches and vomiting had stopped he was still suffering from the aura, or visual disturbances associated with migraine. The report stated that these symptoms usually respond to a small increase in the dose.

Two women in the placebo group were forced to drop out of the test because their migraines returned so severely. One had been taking about 75 mg of dried feverfew powder daily for four and a half years before starting the trial. The other had controlled her migraine successfully with only about 25 mg of dried powder and in the four years before the trial had suffered only two or three attacks a year. When she withdrew from the trial it took longer for the feverfew to relieve the severe problems and the researchers suggest that was because her dosage was only one third of that of the other patient who dropped out. However, eight months after the study, this patient had reduced her dose to only 5 mg and was still free of migraine.

The experiences of the people who were growing feverfew in their gardens and eating fresh raw leaves or drying the leaves to a powder formed the basis for some commercial companies to determine the dosage of their products. Bio-Health makes a 100 mg capsule containing the dried leaf. Managing director David Smith said that when the company started to consider making a feverfew product he drew on his 27 years of experience with a company which supplied practitioners with a liquid extract of feverfew for treating women's complaints and types of arthritis. They were using anything from 3–7 ml of the liquid daily. Bio-Health decided to make dried feverfew rather than a liquid and wanted to produce the equivalent of the lowest liquid dose – 3 ml. When this was calculated for dried feverfew it was found to be the equivalent of 500 mg of dried plants. He reduced this to 100 mg because he was using only the leaf with its extra concentration of sesquiter-pene lactones.

Potters Herbal Supplies markets one of the strongest feverfew tablets on the market at 200 mg. Timothy Whittaker, the company's chief chemist and a registered medical herbalist, states that the 200 mg dose was based on information from users who were growing their own feverfew. These people were eating four small leaves a day, usually in a sandwich to disguise the bitter taste, and they found this amount was effective. Potters examined the amount of dried feverfew from four small leaves and found this was 'pretty close to 200 mg'. Mr Whittaker grows feverfew in his own garden, dries it and pulverises it before putting it into gelatin capsules. He has prescribed both tablets and capsules and he says that the dosage in his home-prepared capsules is nearer 250 mg than Potters 200 mg.

One of his patients tells him that she gets more relief from the pain of her arthritis from his capsules than from other tablets she has taken and he believes that this is due to the higher dosage in his own product. 'It suggests to me that there is scope for investigating higher doses of feverfew than we are using at the moment', he said. However, this is not a view universal among herbalists. Herbalist Claire Swann feels strongly that the dosage should be low. She was particularly upset by a newspaper feature on herbs which advocated taking a heaped teaspoon of dried feverfew and steeping it in a cupful of hot water for fifteen minutes before drinking it as an infusion. She considers that this is far too high a concentration of feverfew and recommends just a level teaspoonful in three-quarters to a pint of water, leaving it to stand for only three to five minutes before drinking.

Claire Swann says that feverfew is one of the more powerful herbs in general use and believes that lower doses can actually be more effective, dismissing the principle that if a little is good a lot will be better. She recommends using the whole herb because she feels that there is more to herbal medicine than just the measurable active ingredients which may one day be isolated and produced synthetically. 'There are forces in herbs which cannot be detected with any instrument', she says. She also feels that using the whole herb is the safest way to treat people, 'even the most dangerous herb has an inbuilt safety device'. However, this is not a belief shared by many scientists.

Mrs Swann uses feverfew in several forms. She has a fluid extract with a suggested dosage of four drops a day in a little water. She believes that taking feverfew regularly over some time will reduce symptoms gradually by building up the body's resistance. When people do get a migraine they can be helped by using feverfew externally in the form of a cream or lotion. She advises people to use these topical preparations in conjunction with the long-term treatment with tincture. A little of the cream or lotion should be rubbed onto the temples, behind the ears and at the seat of the pain to obtain relief.

Because each individual needs careful assessment, her herbal preparations, made from plants grown in her Hampstead garden, are not on general sale, but available only to those who consult her professionally. Treatment varies according to the individual and although she finds feverfew useful in treating migraine in particular and also many other conditions – including skin problems, rheumatic pain, insect bites and melancholia – she keeps an open mind when it comes to choosing herbs to treat each condition and will not necessarily choose feverfew. 'This is where consultation comes in, everyone is different', she says. She offers two further pieces of advice: firstly find out as much as you can about herbs if you are going to grow and use them; secondly, try to dry herbs such as feverfew away from direct heat so that more of the volatile oils containing the active ingredients will be preserved.

Weleda take the low dose principle even further. They produce both a tablet and a liquid prepared homoeo-pathically. Homoeopathy takes a different approach from traditional herbal medicine. The herb is diluted or potentized, producing an infinitesimal dose. By conventional medical standards the amount of the herb in the medicine is barely traceable but homoeopaths say the process of potentization produces a powerful healing force, making it even more effective.

The Weleda products are made to the traditional 6X potency—where the medicine is mixed one part herb to nine parts base material, which in the case of a liquid could be alcohol; then one part of the resulting dilution is mixed with nine parts of the base material and the process goes on until it has been repeated six times. The homoeopathic approach takes two distinctly different lines. One – the so-called classic approach which was developed by homoeopathy's founding father, Samuel Hahneman – uses substances which in a normal strength dose would be poisonous but potentizes them, often more than six times, to stimulate the body's own defence mechanisms against illness. The other approach – and the one which the Weleda feverfew products take – is to use small and therefore, it is argued, more potent doses to subdue symptoms in a more conventional way. This approach has been developed over the years by practising homoeopaths.

The commercially-available feverfew products vary considerably in dosage, in potency, and in the amount of active ingredients contained in them. Different drying or preparation methods result in the loss of different amounts of the volatile oils in which the active constituents are concentrated. While the amount of the herb in a product remains constant, the level of the active ingredients may change from batch to batch. The question of standardizing these ingredients is one which is bound to be pursued more vigorously in future and is discussed later in the book.

Side effects

It is perhaps not surprising that a herb with the power of feverfew should provoke side effects in some people. Users agree that these side effects usually appear very soon after treatment with feverfew is started and soon subside once treatment is stopped. In the report on the City of London Migraine Clinic trial, [3] researchers refer to a questionnaire which Dr Johnson sent to 300 users. Adverse events or side effects were reported by 18 per cent of these people and the most troublesome was mouth ulceration, which was reported by about 11.3 per cent.

Feverfew can also provoke a general soreness and inflammation in the mouth which also affects the tongue and can cause swelling of the lips and even a loss of taste. In the report on the migraine trial the researchers state that these symptoms are distinct from mouth ulceration and may be caused when the leaves are eaten raw – possibly because of the sesquiterpene lactones in the leaves – as the compounds can cause contact dermatitis.

Timothy Whittaker finds that although general mouth soreness may be caused by chewing the leaves, mouth ulcers can arise through taking tablets or capsules as it is not necessary for the feverfew to touch the mouth to cause ulcers. However, he has never had a single patient in his practice who complained of this side effect and he wonders whether some of the people taking commercial products may be reacting to fillers, binders or other substances which may have been added rather than to the feverfew itself.

Some patients may also complain of an itchy skin, possibly accompanied by a rash. One patient testing feverfew for the authors of this book found that within a few days of starting treatment with 200 mg tablets a rash developed on her forehead and her eyes became sore and itchy. The symptoms disappeared within a few days of discontinuing the tablets.

Some women of childbearing age may notice a slight increase in the heaviness of their periods when they start taking feverfew, due no doubt to the herb's traditional ability to induce menstruation and cleanse the womb.

Indigestion or colicky stomach pains have also been reported and a patient trying feverfew for the authors reported a gentle and welcome relief from constipation within a couple of days of starting treatment with 100 mg of dried leaf per day.

As with any treatment, patients who experience side effects should discontinue treatment at once and if symptoms do not disappear within a very few days they should consult their doctor.

CHAPTER 7

Growth, Harvest and Manufacture of Feverfew

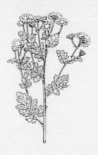

Feverfew was not being grown anywhere on a large scale until the 1980s when it had been sufficiently re-established to be recognized as a viable commercial proposition. Companies developing feverfew products for widespread distribution found that their greatest problem was to locate sufficient supplies of the raw material. Feverfew was only being grown domestically and specialist herb growers could only offer a limited number of plants. The manufacturers had little alternative – they had to grow their own.

Even after making that decision there were still problems to overcome as not all the plants they received for starter stock were the real thing. A great deal of time had to be spent in seeking out growers who could supply genuine *Tanacetum parthenium* rather than other varieties of feverfew, or similar plants from the *Compositae* family such as German chamomile.

The question of how and where to grow it was partially

solved by the decline of the tomato industry in the Channel Islands; a number of growers there were pleased to use their glasshouses to grow feverfew. Among the first companies to investigate the possibilities of producing feverfew commercially were Herbal Laboratories and Potters Herbal Supplies, both based in Lancashire. Both companies have supplies grown in the Channel Islands. Herbal Laboratories also have a major local supplier on the Fylde peninsula which, like the Channel Islands, has a declining market-gardening industry.

This supplier, Stuart Lees, has been a nurseryman all his life. He was the pioneer grower for Herbal Laboratories and is still a major supplier for the company. Growing herbs was a completely new venture for Mr Lees, who had never heard of feverfew until he was approached by Herbal Laboratories. Some of his young workers, however, had read about it in history books and knew it was traditionally known as 'the headache plant'. A supply of plants was obtained from a herb grower in Richmond, Yorkshire, and passed on to Mr Lees for growing and cropping.

In describing how he grows feverfew Stuart Lees says 'The best time to get the best crop is to plant in the spring from March onwards. We sow the seed in blocks with five seeds to the block and then plant out.' He warns potential growers that feverfew is a slow-germinating seed and it can take five or six weeks before a small plant appears. While those first seedlings are establishing themselves more can germinate over the next month. In another month the plants will be large and strong enough to be planted out. 'We grow it in a greenhouse, without extra heat or light,' he said. 'We did try growing it outside, but the weeds overpowered it. For a normal harvest we wait until the plants are two feet high, which takes until mid-July. We harvest before the flowers appear, which is usually when the plant is about three feet high.'

One particular pest is chickweed which can choke the

feverfew plants if left unchecked and the rows of feverfew have to be weeded regularly by hand. 'If the weed gets to be too much of a problem, we have to rotivate it all in and start again,' he said. Grass can also cause trouble if the crop is left in too long. The plants are fed with bone meal and fish blood and bone and the half acre which Mr Lees has put down to the herb could yield an optimum crop of two tons though temperature and weather fluctuations usually reduce that to about one and a half tons.

In a good year the plants can be cropped up to three times and they can be left in the ground for a second year but yield is not generally so good the second time around. Once cut, the herb is spread on long benches in the glasshouses and dried using warm air blowers – a process which can take between three and ten days. 'Like Comfrey, it is full of water, so it is difficult to dry and we get it down to one-tenth of its volume,' he said. Because it is still essentially wild, it is not the easiest plant to grow on a planned commercial basis.

Timothy Whittaker of Potters Herbal Supplies suggested feverfew among a number of items when approached by a Channel Islands tomato and flower grower. The test growing was so successful that Potters asked the grower to supply half a ton of dried feverfew in 1984. The company also took a couple of smaller deliveries from a grower in the Fylde peninsular. The Channel Islands grower dries the herb away from direct sunlight in a glasshouse covered with black polythene.

Bio-Health is another company whose supplies of feverfew are grown in the Channel Islands. Their plants are grown organically.

Some companies have both feverfew and other herbal products made for them under contract but Potters and Herbal Laboratories are among those who make their own and have invested in highly complex analytical equipment which is used in research, development and manufacture. Both carry out routine sampling of bulk herb supplies coming into the factories. Identification tests are crucial, particularly with a herb like feverfew which has so many related species.

Dried feverfew can be made into tablets or capsules and a number of different companies have products on the market. (See chapter 8). Some capsules are filled with pure dried feverfew leaf, others contain the whole herb. Tablets usually contain the whole herb and one of the latest products from Seven Seas (the company best known for its cod liver oil), is covered with a naturally derived coating. Tinctures and essences are made from the freshly-gathered plant or part of the plant by steeping it in alcohol or a mixture of water and alcohol.

CHAPTER 8
Who Makes What?

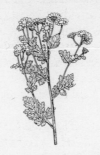

Feverfew is available in a number of forms. It is stocked by health food shops, chemists (particularly those carrying health foods and natural remedies) and by herbalists and practitioners of alternative medicine. If you are unable to find feverfew locally you may like to contact one of the leading suppliers listed here.

Bio-Health Ltd, 13 Oakdale Road, London SW16 2 HP (tel: 01 769 7975). This company produces feverfew capsules under the Pure-Fil label. A bottle contains 60 100 mg capsules of dried feverfew leaf and dosage is one per day.

    Bio-Health promotes its product as being made from organically-grown feverfew, cultivated under contract in the Channel Islands. Allergy sufferers and people sensitive to certain additives are assured that the capsules contain only feverfew leaf with no other substance added. No chemical process is used during manufacture and therefore potential allergens are restricted to the feverfew itself and the hard gelatin capsule in which it is contained.

Booker Health Foods Ltd, Healthways House, 45 Station Approach, West Byfleet, Surrey KT14 6NE (tel: 093 23 41133). Booker market two feverfew preparations. Heath & Heather is a traditional herbal remedy using the whole dried leaf in 25 mg formulation with a recommended dose of two tablets per day. Potter and Clarke offer Lomigran, a product most likely to be found in a chemist's shop, containing a standardized extract of feverfew's active constituents, the sesquiterpene lactones. It comes in capsule form and provides 0.1 mg of the active ingredient, the equivalent of the average amount found in 25 mg of whole, dried feverfew leaf.

Cathay of Bournemouth Ltd, 32 Cleveland Road, Bournemouth, BH1 4QC (tel: 0202 37178). Cathay make feverfew essence from fresh leaves within two hours of picking. One teaspoonful of essence is said to be equivalent to one fresh leaf.

Gerard House (1965) Ltd, 736 Christchurch Road, Bournemouth, Dorset PH7 6BZ (tel: 0202 434116). The company produces Essence of Feverfew in 25 ml bottles. It is made from the fresh herb within two hours of harvesting and subjected to a cold process of maceration in water and alcohol which acts as a preserving agent and solvent. Dosage is five drops to be taken three times daily between meals.

The Health & Diet Food Company Ltd, Seymour House, South Street, Godalming, Surrey GU7 1BZ (tel: 04868 28021). Super Feverfew from Health & Diet is marketed under its Food Supplement Company (FSC) brand. This 150 mg tablet in packs of 60 is one of the newest feverfew products to come on to the market.

Herbal Laboratories Ltd, Copse Road, Fleetwood,

Lancashire FY7 7PF (tel: 03917 70027). The company produces bottles of 30 or 90 125 mg tablets containing the whole dried herb. Dosage is one tablet daily.

Lifeplan Products Ltd, Elizabethan Way, Lutterworth, Leicestershire ME17 4ND (tel: 04555 56461). This company makes 250 mg dried leaf capsules under the Natural Selection brand name.

A. Nelson & Co Ltd, 5 Endeavour Way, Wimbledon, London SW19 9UH (tel: 01 946 8527). Nelsons offer feverfew in extract form in a 50 ml dropper bottle. Dosage is five drops in a tablespoon of water night and morning. The whole fresh flowering plant is used to prepare the tincture which contains alcohol.

Potter's (Herbal Supplies) Ltd, Leyland Mill Lane, Wigan, Lancashire WN1 25B (tel: 0942 34761/5). Under the Barefoot Brand the company offers 200 mg tablets in packs of 30 or 90. Dosage is one tablet daily. A three-month course is recommended.

Power Health Products Ltd, 10 Central Avenue, Airfield Estate, Pocklington, York YO4 2NR (tel: 07592 2595/2734). The company offers 200 mg capsules made from feverfew grown and dried in the South of France. No fillers or binders are added.

Seven Seas Health Care Ltd, Hedon Road, Marfleet, Hull HU9 5NJ (tel: 0482 75234). The company produces feverfew as one of a range of herbal remedies launched in 1986. The 100 mg coated tablets come in boxes of 30 with a recommended dosage of one tablet daily.

Weleda (UK) Ltd, Heanor Road, Ilkeston, Derbyshire DE7 8DR (tel: 0602 309319). Weleda have two feverfew products, both prepared to the standard homoeopathic 6X potency. One or two tablets are recommended to be taken daily for six weeks. The suggested dose for the liquid preparation is five drops twice a day. Weleda drops are suitable for vegans.

CHAPTER 9

Growing Your Own

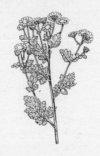

There are many users of feverfew who still say that no matter how good commercial products are there is nothing as good as fresh leaves picked from the garden. Feverfew is an easy herb to grow at home – indeed it may already be flourishing in your garden without you realizing that it is anything more than a persistent and attractive interloper. It will even grow in poor soil but appreciates being planted in a semi-shaded spot. It does not need special attention to survive but young plants should not be choked by weeds. The seeds may germinate slowly and haphazardly and, typical of a wild plant, more seedlings will be produced long after the first ones have appeared.

Although hardy enough to be grown outdoors feverfew can be potted and brought inside. Folklore maintains that its presence indoors will help to ward off headaches. One company making feverfew products quotes an old country-man from Shropshire who said 'Keep feverfew in 'ouse and you'll never get 'eadache.'

Mrs Jenkins, who has years of experience of growing and

preserving feverfew, has given advice to hundreds of back-garden feverfew growers. We pass on some of her tips:

Keep several plants but allow only one to flower to provide the seeds for new plants. Flower heads from the others should be removed.

During the winter bring four or five plants into the greenhouse or cover them with a cloche to preserve them from the worst of the frost.

Anyone who wants to continue taking fresh feverfew whilst away from home can keep cut leaves fresh for a short while by immersing the cut stems in water. Feverfew can be dried and preserved for those who want to make sure that their supply does not dry up in winter.

Leaves should be picked at the height of the growing season in the summer on a dry day; leaves which are damp tend to deteriorate and lose their potency. The leaves should be clean and free from insecticides. Once gathered they should be dried and this is an important process in which moisture is removed from the herb. Feverfew is full of moisture and will lose 75–82 per cent of its original weight when dry. A typical dose of one large or three small leaves, as recommended by Mrs Jenkins, will yield only one heaped saltspoonful when dried and ground by hand.

When drying leaves it is important not to wash them after collection but to spread them singly on a muslin covered tray in shady, airy conditions at a temperature of not more than 40°C (104°F), for example in an airing cupboard. Frequent turning will help to ensure that the leaves are dried thoroughly and the process should take three to four days. When the leaves are properly dried they can be hand ground, powdered and stored in a screwtop jar away from the light.

Mrs Jenkins says that one heaped saltspoonful of fever-few can be mixed with a little honey and spread on bread or toast and this is a fairly easy way to take the daily dose.

If you want to start growing feverfew for medicinal use it

is vital to obtain the right plants. If you cannot obtain the genuine article from a friend's garden you should go to a reputable grower. The Herb Society may be able to supply a list of growers and the authors offer the following list of feverfew suppliers.

John Chambers, 15 Westleigh Road, Barton Seagrave, Kettering, Northants NN15 5AJ. Mr Chambers supplies seeds and plants and will send a catalogue listing prices and availability if you write enclosing a stamped, self-addressed envelope.

Yorkshire Herbs, The Herb Centre, Middleton Tyas, Richmond, North Yorkshire DL10 6RR, offer plants and some dried leaf.

Hollington Nurseries Ltd, Woolton Hill, Newbury, Berks RG15 9XP, sell feverfew plants.

Suffolk Herbs, Sawyers Farm, Little Canard, Sudbury, Suffolk CO10 0NY, sells seeds.

CHAPTER 10
Where to From Here?

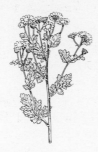

Numerous people will testify to the fact that feverfew works for them but this is not enough to satisfy the scientific and medical establishment. Testimonial evidence, however strong and however extensive, will never satisfy doctors and scientists who are unsympathetic to what they see as crank or fringe medicines and who take a more dispassionate view than the enthusiasts whose delight at relief from pain and discomfort may colour their judgement.

Satisfied users of feverfew will continue to take it whether migraine specialists, rheumatologists, GPs and research scientists approve or not but if feverfew is to reach its full potential and to become available for a wider public then scientific appraisal is a necessary part of the way forward. Although the scientific work done so far has produced some encouraging and positive results for feverfew, much more work needs to be done. More studies into both migraine and arthritis need to be made. As yet no clinical trials involving arthritis patients have been completed and the clinical trial at the City of London Migraine Clinic, [3] which was given great prominence in the media, did in fact only involve 17 patients. Data from this trial has been seized upon as it is the only evidence of its kind currently available and there is always a danger that when such evidence is presented in popular form the public may assume that the case for feverfew has been proven and nothing further needs to be done.

The results certainly demonstrate that feverfew can prevent or lessen migraine. The patients in each group were able to guess accurately whether they were taking the real thing or dummy capsules and the fact that two people were so ill without feverfew that they had to drop out of the trials is in itself an argument for using the herb medicinally. But the research team themselves stress the need for tests involving many more patients to add further weight to the case. There should be no shortage of patients willing to take part in trials as any request for testimonial evidence from feverfew users is greeted with a positive avalanche of response.

Clinical trials involving arthritis patients will be particularly interesting as the only study which has been published in the UK as far as we are aware was a laboratory test using blood. The results demonstrate the various ways in which feverfew is active and throw new light on how it might interfere with the course of rheumatoid arthritis, as well as its possible effects on migraine and psoriasis. Osteoarthritis and often unspecified rheumatic aches and pains were not accounted for, though there are many people who find relief from these conditions by using the herb. There may be several more areas in which feverfew may be used which have not been investigated scientifically where reports have been made of unexpected beneficial side effects such as alleviation of hay fever or tension.

Manufacturers are concerned that the real value and reputation of the herb should not be undermined by extravagant claims for it as a cure-all. New research could be made into its effects on the central nervous system, on stress, hay fever, insect bites, gynaecological problems, psoriasis and other skin troubles. More work could also be done to look at the active ingredients and to find out whether those sesquiterpene lactones which are present only in tiny amounts also have an important role to play. The wide choice of doses among commercial products and the lack of control over amounts of raw herb leave dosage as an open question. Views vary on the most efficacious dose but no comparative tests have been made.

John Grady of Herbal Laboratories believes that testimonial evidence on a wide enough scale can be valuable, especially if clinical evidence is limited. He has provided feverfew tablets for a trial conducted among readers of *Here's Health* magazine. Sufferers from arthritis, migraine and other ailments, who had not tried feverfew were invited to send for a course of tablets and to report on the results. The test was just starting at the time of writing this book but it was hoped that at least 2000 people would take part. Mr Grady does not have any misgivings about tests on feverfew and would be happy to co-operate in any controlled clinical trials. He believes that the experiences from unsupervised self-treatment should not be undervalued. 'For things like migraine and arthritis, testimonial evidence is important because the results are measurable. With arthritis it is possible to see that joints which were once swollen are no longer so and again, with migraine, if someone has regularly had attacks over a number of years and then no longer has them, it is something else which is quantifiable.'

A standard feverfew?

Because the whole herb or parts of the whole herb are used in commercial preparations, the amount of active in-

gredient varies from plant to plant, batch to batch and
season to season. Some manufacturers have investigated the
possibility of producing a feverfew tablet or capsule
containing a standard amount of the active ingredient – the
sesquiterpene lactones. Even this can give rise to difficulty as
there are many different sesquiterpene lactones in feverfew,
with different degrees of activity. Until further examination
has revealed the parts played by the individual substances it
will be this group of chemicals which will be used as the
basis for standardization.

Dr John Pugh considers that extraction of parthenolide,
believed to be the most important of the sesquiterpene
lactones, would be relatively simple. It is concentrated in
small glands on the underside of the leaves and to rupture
them and to collect the parthenolide as it is released would
be an easy process. He has found that the parthenolide
content in feverfew diminishes as the plant matures.

Standardization is not a policy which all companies will
be adopting. Timothy Whittaker of Potters said that to get a
standard amount of sesquiterpene lactones in all the tablets
it may be necessary to vary the amount of herb in the
product as the sesquiterpene lactone content of each batch
of raw material would vary. An alternative method of
standardization would be to extract the active ingredient
from the herbal material and put that into a product. He
believes that this may not be satisfactory as the extracted
sesquiterpene lactone may not be as stable as when it is in
the leaf with the result that the product could have a very
short shelf life.

R. P. Scherer is one pharmaceutical company which is
convinced that there is a future for a product with a
guaranteed consistent level of active ingredients. It has
already developed Lomigran, a standardized feverfew
which is being marketed in the UK by Potter and Clarke, a
Booker Health Foods company. Scherer have also received

a number of inquiries from interested European companies. Lomigran is standardized on the entire sesquiterpene lactone content. Although parthenolide is the sesquiterpene lactone known to play a significant part in feverfew's activity, scientists believe that further tests may show that other constituents also have an important role.

Synthetic feverfew?

When a herbal material has been shown to be successful – and existing work indicates feverfew as a potential candidate – science may wish to attempt to reproduce it synthetically. A synthetic product eliminates the supply problems often experienced by herbal manufacturers and for those making feverfew. It is unlikely, however, that a synthetic drug based on feverfew's active ingredients will be available in the near future. Much analytical work remains to be done and extensive safety tests would have to be passed. In the opinion of Dr Pugh synthesizing the active ingredient would be difficult because parthenolide, for example, is a highly complex molecule. Herbalists present a strong case for using the whole herb and not something out of a test tube. They believe that any active ingredient is more effectively administered in its natural state than when it is isolated for use and the sum of all the active ingredients taken individually is much smaller than when they are acting together in the whole herb.

Feverfew and the Medicines Act

Feverfew is not officially recognized as a medicine and without a product licence under the Medicines Act it has to be sold as a food supplement. The 1968 Medicines Act was introduced after the Thalidomide tragedy to try to prevent potentially harmful medicines from coming on to the market. When the Act came into force medicines already on sale with a long safety record were granted licences 'of right'. In order to sell a new product with medicinal claims companies are required to obtain a product licence from the DHSS. Licences are only granted after lengthy, wide-ranging and costly clinical trials. Herbal manufacturers say this puts them at a disadvantage because they lack the assets of the multinational drug companies. However, since they deal with plants which are commonly available and are not creating new drugs, they may sell their products as food supplements – provided that they do not make claims for them and provided that they are not poisonous. They may therefore produce what it is in effect a medicinal product and taken as such by the public without having to adhere to the rules governing official medicines.

This situation is unsatisfactory both for the manufacturer who is unable to make claims for his products and for the consumer who must rely on the knowledge and experience of those selling the goods for advice.

The DHSS is carrying out a long overdue review of the licences granted 'of right', and reassessing the acceptability and safety of products sold as medicines. Manufacturers have united to form the Natural Medicines Group and are trying to influence the government's attitude towards herbal medicine. They are pressing for experts in herbal medicine to be appointed to the review body to advise on herbal products and they are proposing that testimonial evidence on a large scale should be an acceptable assessment of the efficacy of herbal medicines in the absence of clinical evidence.

If the government does agree to this many more products would be included under the licensing system. Manu-facturers, most of whom currently produce unlicensed products to the same high standard as for licensed medicines, maintain that this could only have positive results through stricter quality regulation.

Health food shop or prescription?

This question was posed by the *Lancet* [1] in its comment on the Nottingham findings:

> When the active principle responsible for this activity is identified (and feverfew contains several potential candidates in addition to the sesquiterpene lactone, parthenolide) will such an identification transform feverfew from a health food, which any member of the public can grow or buy without medical, pharmaceutical, or chemical advice, into a drug? Will regulatory bodies then require many years of laboratory and animal studies before it can be moved back into the patients with arthritis, migraine and psoriasis who are currently consuming it without any advice or supervision? If so, patients will surely put pressure on the medical profession to get on with trials of herbal tablets of known source and potency rather than to embark on a search for the chemical identity of the active principle.

Certainly, it would be regrettable if steps were taken to restrict the availability of feverfew. Indeed it is difficult to see how this could be done with any measure of success since it is grown domestically. There is no doubt that removal of feverfew products from the shelves of health food shops would be unpopular and grossly unfair considering the industry's role in fostering renewed interest in the herb.

Sources

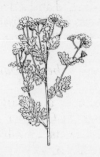

[1] 'Feverfew' – A New Drug or an Old Wives' Remedy?, the *Lancet* (11 May 1985).

[2] Culpeper, Nicholas, *Complete Herbal* (Omega Books, 1985).

[3] Johnson, Dr E. S. et al., 'Efficacy of Feverfew as Prophylactic Treatment of Migraine', *The British Medical Journal*, vol. 291 (31 August 1985).

[4] Hylands, Dr D. M., 'How to identify the correct variety of feverfew', *Migraine Matters*, vol. 2, no. 4 (October–December 1984).

[5] Bancke's Herball, an anonymous work published in 1525 by printer Richard Bancke. Arber, Agnes, Herbals! Then Origins and Evolution 1470–1670, Cambridge University 1938.

[6] Gerard, John, *The Herball or General Historie of Plantes* (1597, rev. 1927 as *Leaves from Gerard's Herball*, ed. Marcus Woodward).

[7] Hill MD, Sir John, *The Family Herbal* (Bungay, 1812).

[8] Chapman, Robert, 'Weed sandwiches end a wife's migraine', *Sunday Express* (1978).

[9] Heptinstall, Dr S. et al., 'Extracts of Feverfew Inhibit Granule Secretion in Blood Platelets and Polymorphonuclear Leucocytes', the *Lancet* (11 May 1985).

[10] Drozda, B. and Bloszyk, E., *Planta Medica* 1978.

[11] Bohlmann, Ferdinand and Zdera, Christa, 'Sesqutiterpene Lactones and other Constituents from Tanacetum Parthenium', *Phytochemistry* vol. 21, no. 10, (1982), pp. 2543–9.

[12] Hylands, Dr P. J., *The Herbal Review*, vol. 8, no. 3 (summer, 1983).

[13] Hanington, Edda et al., 'Migraine: A Platelet Disorder', the *Lancet* (3 October 1981).

[14] Migraine, The Facts, published by The British Migraine Association.

[15] Mills, Simon Y., *The Dictionary of Modern Herbalism* (Thorsons Publishing Group, 1985).

[16] Wood, Philip H. N. and Badley, Elizabeth M., *If You've Got Arthritis Expert Advice is Badly Needed* (The Arthritis and Rheumatism Council, 1983 [a report on a survey of the availability of specialist rheumatologists]). *Introducing Arthritis*, an Arthritis and Rheumatism Council patient handbook, published 1986.

[17] Woodward, Dr Elizabeth, 'Feverfew – Many Uses and Forms', *The Herbal Review* (winter, 1980).

[18] Berry, Dr M. I., 'Feverfew Faces the Future', *The Pharmaceutical Journal* (19 May 1984).

ADDITIONAL READING

Bailey, J. Martyn and Makheja A. N., 'The Active Principle in Feverfew, the *Lancet* (7 November 1981).

Bartram FNIMH, T., 'Feverfew', *Grace Magazine*.

Howe, G. B. and Fordham J. N., 'Polymorphonuclear

Leucocytes, Origins, Functions and Roles in the Rheumatic Diseases' in W. Carson Dick (ed.) *Immunological Aspects of Rheumatology* (Lancaster MTP Press, 1981).

Jenkins, Ann, 'Feverfew' *Welsh Medical Gazette* (September 1985).

Le Strange, Richard, *A History of Herbal Plants* (Angus & Robertson Publishers, 1977).

Scott, J. T., *Arthritis and Rheumatism The Facts* (Oxford University Press, 1980).

Stuart, Malcolm (ed.), *Encyclopaedia of Herbs and Herbalism* (Orbis Publishing Ltd, 1979).

Tortora, Gerard J. and Anagnostakos, Nicholas P., *Principles of Anatomy and Physiology* (New York: Harper & Row, 1984).

Wilkinson, Dr Marcia, 'Migraine & Headaches', in Martin Dunitz, *Positive Health Guide* (1982).

Useful addresses

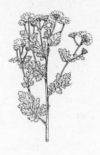

The British Migraine Association, 178a High Road, Byfleet, Weybridge, Surrey KT14 7ED.

The City of London Migraine Clinic, 22 Charterhouse Square, London EC1M 6DX.

The Herb Society, 34 Boscobel Place, London SW1W 9PE.

Index

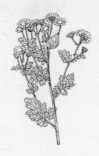

Dictionary of Modern
      Herbalism 20, 35
dosage 41–45, 61

Fylde Peninsular 41, 50

Gerard House (1965) Ltd 53
Gerard, John 6, 35, 37
Grady, John 13, 61
gynaecological conditions 5,
      6, 24, 34–35, 39, 42,
      46

Haddington, Edda 17
Hancock, Ken 10–11, 14
hay fever 36–37, 60
Health & Diet Food Company
      Ltd 53
Heath & Heather 53
Heptinstall, Dr Stan 14, 18
Herbal Laboratories Ltd 13,
      49, 50, 53, 61
Herbal Review 15, 34
Herb Society 58
Here's Health magazine 61
high blood pressure 40
Hill, Sir John 7
Hollington Nurseries 58
Hylands, Dr Deborah (née
      Jessup) 4, 12, 15, 21
Hylands, Dr Peter 11, 15, 16,
      21

insect bites 5, 6, 37–38, 44

Jenkins, Ann 9, 10, 11, 19,
      24–26, 36, 41, 56–57

Johnson, Dr Stewart 16, 21,
      36, 45

Kadam, N. P. 21

Lancet 12, 17, 18, 30, 31, 65
Lees, Stuart 49–50
Liddell, Jo 20, 40
Lifeplan Products Ltd 54
Linsley, Joan 31–32, 34
Lomigran 53, 62, 63

Medicines Act, 1968 9, 63–64
migraine 4, 5, 9, 10, 11, 12,
      15, 16, 17, 18, 19–29,
      30, 31, 44, 59, 61
Mills, Simon 20, 35, 37

National Institute of Medical
      Herbalists 20
Natural Medicines Group 64
A. Nelson & Co Ltd 54
Non-steroidal anti-
      inflammatory drugs 18

parthenolide 15, 16, 62, 63
Pharmaceutical Journal, The
      37
platelets 16, 17, 18
Plutarch 5
polymorphonuclear leucocytes
      17, 18
Potter and Clarke 53, 62
Potters (Herbal Supplies) Ltd
      13, 42, 43, 49, 50, 54,
      62